APPLE CIDER VINEGAR
REMEDIES

TABLE OF CONTENTS

INTRODUCTION

Apple cider vinegar (ACV), which is commonly referred to as ACV, is a type of vinegar used as a natural remedy and also as an ingredient in salad dressings. This type of vinegar, especially organic ACV, is nutrient-rich and is used to control weight loss, blood levels, among other uses. Foods such as oranges, maple syrup, grapes, etc. are used in the production of some kinds of vinegar, all of which have their unique benefits and specific flavors. In the production of ACV, some specific bacteria act on fermented apple juice and convert the liquid to vinegar. The sweet and crispy flavor of the apple cider vinegar is as a result of the compounds in the apples.

The beauty of this vinegar is its versatility; it could be used in many ways, giving you several opportunities to experiment with it in your daily meal plan. For example, you can incorporate ACV into your breakfast, lunch, dinner, and even snacking in between. It can also be added to smoothies to boost the taste and can be drizzled over your salad so as to give it a unique flavor and as a healthier substitute. You can as well glaze your meat dishes with apple cider vinegar combined with other lean ingredients to tweak to your recipe.

The numerous health benefits that are associated with the use of apple cider vinegar are further discussed in subsequent chapters of this book.

CHAPTER 1: ABOUT APPLE CIDER VINEGAR

Apple cider vinegar is known in the natural health community to be the most common type of vinegar. It is gotten from fermented apple liquid and popularly used in vinaigrettes, marinades, salad dressings, food preservatives, , and chutneys. It is found to possess several healing properties, most of which have been validated by science. In the making of apple cider vinegar, apples are crushed and then juiced. The benefits associated with this type of vinegar include but not limited to; weight loss, reduced cholesterol, blood sugar level control, and improved symptoms of diabetes. Also, apple cider vinegar has various household, beauty, and cooking uses that include cleaning, hair washing, food preservation, care of the immune system, and skin function. Several studies that have been carried out on this type of vinegar revealed that it can increase satiety and help the user consume lesser calories, which invariably results in weight loss. When vinegar is taken together with a meal high in carbohydrate, there will be an increased sense of fullness, which eventually leads to less calorie consumption for the rest of that day. It is, however, pertinent to be cautious when applying Apple cider vinegar on the skin. This is because there is tendency for reactions (major skin irritation) such as burns or blisters when it is applied topically without any dilution. The acid in the apple cider vinegar helps to alter pH levels of the skin and ensures good skincare. ACV is effective in attacking the fungus/bacteria causing bad odor and therefore help to diminish the odor. It is very rich in vitamins and minerals, and this makes it a functional ingredient for hair and skincare.

Healing Properties and Benefits of ACV

1. ACV has healing properties that fights against bacterial, fungal and viral infections. This implies that diseases caused by bacteria, fungus and virus can be treated using apple cider vinegar. Some of these diseases include candida, ear infections, allergies, ulcers, acne, etc.

2. ACV helps in weight reduction. It is no news that there are ailments and health risks associated with being overweight. This can be managed with the help of apple cider vinegar. Acetic acid, which is a significant component of ACV, is known to help in weight loss and weight management.

3. ACV is an excellent remedy for diabetes. This type of vinegar has enormous positive effect on blood and insulin levels. This makes it an excellent natural remedy choice for diabetic patients as it is able to help in improving the serum lipid profile and insulin sensitivity of people fighting diabetes.

4. ACV also helps to manage cancer. The acetic acid in ACV is said to have the ability to kill cancer cells by merely starving the cells of the energy required for them to develop. This quality makes ACV a good natural remedy for cancer prevention and management.

5. Apple cider vinegar generally helps to improve digestion and relief stomach problems; it also aids the immune system and improves the condition of the human body (the hair, skin, etc.)

Side Effects of Apple Cider Vinegar

Research had found that ACV has numerous health benefits. Nevertheless, taking too much of vinegar may result it unwanted effects. The following are the possible adverse effects of using excess of apple cider vinegar:

Tooth Decay

People may get tooth decay if they eat too much of acidic foods. ACV is acidic, just like all other vinegar. Taking too much of acidic beverages and foods will lessen the strength of the tooth enamel overtime and can eventually lead to tooth decay.

According to the National Institute of Dental and Craniofacial Research, people might not realize initially, the damaged of their tooth enamel. As the damage gets worse, they begin to experience ache in the teeth or become sensitive to sweet food and cold or hot temperature. Ultimately, the teeth might develop cavities that require fillings. Consuming undiluted ACV regularly tends to increase the risk of getting tooth decay. Taking vinegar as only part of a meal or diluting it reduces the risk.

Gastrointestinal Issues

Apple cider vinegar, ACV, is recommended by many people as a natural weight loss aid. Study established that it helps to slow the rate at which food leaves the stomach, which suppresses the desire for food by making the consumer feels fuller for a long period. Nevertheless, keeping food in the stomach may result in some side effects. In a study conducted to investigate the possibility of ACV to control the desire for food, several participants reported feelings of indigestion and nausea after taking it with breakfast. Due to the acidity, consuming undiluted ACV could also aggravate symptoms in those that have digestives issues, such as acid reflux or ulcers.

Skin Burns

The acidity of apple cider vinegar implies that applying undiluted ones directly to the skin may result in irritation and burns. The National Capital Center list several medical reports where people got severe burns that needed medical attention after applying vinegar directly to their skin.

Safe Usage Tips

Frequently taking large amounts of undiluted vinegar (whether drinking it or leaving it on the skin for long) may cause unwanted side effects. So, to reduce the side effects of ACV:

- Reduce the amount of ACV consumed

- Reduce the number of times you apply ACV to your skin

- Use ACV as an ingredient or dilute with water

- Avoid or limit contact with the teeth, for example, you can drink ACV using a straw

A review in 2016 suggested that people can achieve most of the potential health benefits of vinegar by drinking about 15ml of it daily or any quantity that has about 750mg of acetic acid.

Nevertheless, due to the insufficient research into long-term safety and side effects, the best approach is further moderation.

People with diabetes, low potassium levels or digestive problems should try to consult a physician before taking ACV

A person that experience serious side effects should consult a medical professional.

CHAPTER 2: APPLE CIDER VINEGAR FOOD AND DRINK RECIPES

ACV Salad Dressing

Ingredients:

- 1 small shallot (peeled, cored and quartered)
- ⅓ cup of extra-virgin olive oil
- ¼ cup of cider vinegar
- 2 tsp of honey
- 2 tsp of Dijon mustard
- Salt and pepper to taste

Instructions:

- Puree the shallot, olive oil, vinegar, mustard, honey, salt, and pepper in a blender. Do this for about 30 seconds until the mix is smooth.

- Use immediately or store recipe in a well-sealed jar and put in the refrigerator for up to 1 week.

- Bring recipe back to room temperature before serving if it becomes solid.

ACV Citrus Dill Vinaigrette

Ingredients

- 3 tbsp of fresh lemon juice

- 1 tbsp of cider vinegar

- ¼ cup of extra virgin olive oil

- ½ tsp of dried dill

- Salt to taste

- Black pepper to taste

- Sugar to taste

- ½ tbsp of Dijon mustard

Instructions:

- Whisk all ingredients together in a small mixing bowl until well-blended.

- Taste for salt/pepper and add more if needed. Then, cover the bowl and refrigerate until ready to use. Remember to shake well before using.

ACV Healthy Ketchup

Ingredients:

- 1 tsp of Chia seeds for thickening (optional)

- 36 oz. jar of organic tomato paste

- ½ cup of apple cider vinegar

- 1 tsp of garlic powder

- 1 tbsp of onion powder

- ½ tsp of stevia powder or honey

- 2 tbsp of molasses

- 1 tsp of sea salt

- 1 tsp of mustard powder

- 1 pinch of cinnamon cloves

- 1 pinch of allspice

- 1 pinch of cayenne

- 1 cup of water

Instruction:

- Grind the Chia seeds in a blender or process the seeds in a food processor on high speed for 30 seconds until finely powdered.

- Add all the remaining ingredients to the blender and blend on high speed for about 2 to 3 minutes or use the food processor.

- Transfer into an airtight quart jar and refrigerate for 2 hours or better still, refrigerate overnight to let flavors blend.

* Store in the refrigerator until you are ready to use

ACV Grapefruit Juice

Ingredients:

* 1 cup of fresh grapefruit juice

* 2 tbsp of unfiltered apple cider vinegar

* 1 tsp of honey to taste (optional)

* Ice (optional)

Instructions:

* Make fresh grapefruit juice either by using a juicer or by squeezing the juice out.

* Combine the grapefruit juice together with the apple cider vinegar in a glass and stir.

* Taste the combination and add honey or sweetener if you so desire. Serve directly in a glass or over ice.

ACV Tomato Cider

Ingredients:

- 1 cup of Clean Water

- ½ cup of Tomato Juice

- 2 tbsp of Apple Cider Vinegar

- Pinch of salt (optional)

- Ice

Instructions:

- Simply mix all the ingredients together and serve.

ACV Sweet Juice

Ingredients:

- ½ Teaspoon Sugar

- 2 dashes of bitters

- 4 oz apple cider vinegar

- 3 oz bourbon

- Apple Slices for garnishes (if desired)

- 4 ice cubes

Instructions

- In a glass, add the ½ tsp of sugar and dashes of bitters. Stir together to dissolve the sugar

- Then pour in the cider vinegar, bourbon and add the ice cubes

- Stir well to combine

- Garnish recipe with fresh apple slice(s) if desired

- Serve and enjoy

ACV Cranberry Cocktail

Ingredients:

- 2 Tbsp of cider vinegar

- 2 Tbsp of cranberry juice

- 2 tsp of maple syrup

- 1 ½ cups of water

Instructions:

- Put together all the ingredients in a glass

- Stir and enjoy

ACV Detox Drink

Ingredients:

- 1 cup of water

- 2 tbsp of apple cider vinegar

- 1 teaspoon of freshly grated ginger

- 2 tbsp of freshly squeezed lemon juice

- ¼ teaspoon of ground cinnamon

- 1 teaspoon of raw honey (optional)

- Dash of cayenne pepper

Instructions:

- Boil the water in a saucepan, turn off the heat when boiled, and allow the water to cool a bit. After that, put together all the ingredients. Stir and allow it to steep for a couple of minutes.

- Filter the detox drink into your favorite glass and drink.

Limeade apple cider vinegar drink

Ingredients:

- 1 ½ tbsp of apple cider vinegar

- 1 tbsp of fresh lime juice

- 1 teaspoon of stevia

- 2 cups of cold water

Instructions:

- Mix all the ingredients together

- Serve cold

Ginger Spice Apple Cider Vinegar Drink

Ingredients:

- 1 tbsp of apple cider vinegar

- 1 teaspoon of stevia

- ¼ tsp of ground ginger

- 2 cups of cold water

Instructions:

- Combine all the ingredients together

- Serve cold

ACV Apple Drink

Ingredients:

- 1 tablespoon of apple cider vinegar

- 2 tablespoons of organic apple juice

- ¼ teaspoon of ground cinnamon

- 2 cups of cold water

Instructions:

- Combine all the ingredients together

- Serve cold

ACV Honey Cayenne Drink

Ingredients:

- 1 tbsp of apple cider vinegar

- 1 dash of cayenne pepper

- 2 tbsp of honey (preferably raw & local)

- 2 cups of warm/hot water

Instructions:

- Combine all ingredients until the honey has dissolved. Serve warm or store in the fridge to chill.

ACV Chicken Adobo

Ingredients:

- 2 lb. of skin-on, bone-in chicken thighs

- 2/3 cup of apple cider vinegar

- 1/3 cup of tamari or soy sauce

- 12 garlic cloves (peeled and smashed)

- 2 bay leaves

- 1 tsp of coarsely ground black pepper

- Salt

- Steamed white rice (if desired)

Instructions:

- Prepare a sizable instant pot, about 6-quart. Put the chicken thighs in it (with the skin side down)

- Add in the vinegar, soy sauce or tamari, garlic cloves, black pepper, and the bay leaves.

- Ensure the lid on the instant pot is secured and the valve is in the sealing position as well. Now set the instant pot to pressure cook on high for about 15minutes. Do not force the instant pot to release its pressure but allow the pot to naturally release its pressure. Then, line a baking sheet that's rimmed with aluminum foil and place a rack in the middle of the oven.

- Use tongs to open the instant pot and transfer the chicken to the lined baking sheet skin-side up. Set aside.

- Press the Sauté button on the instant pot and set timer to run for 10minutes while frequently stirring. Mash the cloves in the sauce with a wooden spoon if desired.

- Broil the chicken in the oven until it becomes nicely browned (rotate the baking sheet as required).

- Taste the sauce and adjust the seasoning with salt and additional pepper if required. (Dispose the bay leaves)

- Serve the chicken thighs. Ladle the sauce over the chicken and enjoy with rice.

ACV Keto Shepherd Pie

Ingredients:

- 1 medium head cauliflower, cut into florets (about 6 cups)

- 4 oz of cream cheese, softened

- ¼ cup of heavy cream

- 1 ½ cup of shredded cheddar, divided

- 2 green onions, thinly sliced

- Kosher salt

- Freshly ground black pepper

- 1 tbsp. extra-virgin olive oil

- 1 small yellow onion (chopped)

- 1 medium carrot (peeled and chopped)

- 3 garlic cloves (minced)

- 1 tbsp. of tomato paste

- 1 pound of ground beef

- ½ cup of low-sodium beef broth

Instructions:

- Heat up oven to a temperature of 400°. Add water and salt to a large pot and bring to a boil. Add cauliflower florets and cook for about 10 minutes until tender. Drain off excess water using a clean dish towel or paper towels.

- Return cauliflower to the pot, add cream cheese and mash the cauliflower using a potato masher until smooth.

- Then add in the heavy cream with 1 cup of cheddar and half of the green onions. Stir well to combine and add salt and pepper to taste.

- Heat oil in a prepared skillet over medium heat. Add onion and carrots to the skillet and cook until soft.

This should take about 5 minutes. Then add garlic and cook until aroma is released.

- Afterwards, add the tomato paste and mix well to coat veggies. Add ground beef to the mixture in the skillet. Break the meat using a wooden spoon and cook for about 6 minutes until it's no longer pink. Season with salt and pepper, add broth and simmer for about 2 minutes.

- Place the cauliflower mash inside the skillet, then top with remaining ½ cup of cheddar. Bake until the top is golden and cheese is melted, 20 minutes.

- Top with more green onions to serve.

ACV Beet-pickled Deviled Eggs

Ingredients:

- 6 large eggs

- 1 can of pickled beets

- 1 cup of cider vinegar

- 1/3 cup of packed brown sugar

- 1 tbsp of peppercorn

- 1 tsp of salt (add more if needed)

- 2 tbsp of Olive oil

- I tbsp of mayonnaise

- 1 tbsp of distilled white vinegar

- 1 tsp of Dijon mustard

- ½ tsp of curry powder

- Freshly ground black pepper

- Chopped fresh rosemary leaves (for garnish)

Instructions:

- Boil eggs and remove the egg shells.

- Pour a can of pickled beets into a sizable mixing bowl to prepare the brine. Stir in the apple cider vinegar, sugar, salt and peppercorns. Gently and carefully place the peeled eggs into the prepared brine. Cover and refrigerate for a minimum of 12 hours or for as long as 3 days. The longer they are left in the brine, the sourer and pinker they become.

- When the brining time is completed, remove the eggs from the brine. Cut each egg in half from top to bottom. Scoop out the yolks and place in a medium bowl. After that, add the olive oil, mayonnaise, white vinegar, mustard, and curry powder. Mix and mash using a fork until smooth. Add little water to the mixture if the mix is too stiff. And then, season with salt and pepper to taste.

- Scoop all the filling into a re-sealable sandwich bag using a scapula. Press the bag with hands to push the filling to one corner and press any air out of the top. (If using a plastic bag, snip off one corner of the bag with a pair of scissors.)

- Pipe filling into the cup of each egg white, filling the cups so that the filling mounds a little over the top. Squeeze the bag from the top to force the mixture downward. (Alternatively, scoop the filling into the egg whites with a spoon.) Drizzle with chopped rosemary and season with salt and pepper.

ACV Beet Salad with Bacon

Ingredients:

- 1 lb of golden beets, peeled and cut into wedges

- 2 center-cut bacon slices

- 1 cup of sliced red onion

- 2 tbsp of apple cider vinegar

- 1/4 tsp of black pepper

- 1 tbsp of chopped fresh chives

Instructions:

- Wrap beets in microwave-safe parchment paper. Microwave until tender, about 11 to 12 minutes.

- Cook bacon in a skillet over medium-high heat until crisp. Once done, drain it on paper towels and reserve drippings in pot. Crumble the bacon. After that, add onion to pot and cook for two minutes. Remove pot from heat. Stir in vinegar and pepper, add beets and then toss. Sprinkle with bacon and chives.

ACV Pan Roasted Vegetables

Ingredients

- 3 tbsp of olive oil

- 1 tbsp of freshly chopped thyme

- 2 tbsp of whole-grain mustard

- 1 tbsp of cider vinegar, divided

- ¾ tsp of kosher salt

- 3 cups of peeled, chopped butternut squash

- ½ tsp of ground black pepper (fresh)

- 1 lb of parsnips, (peeled and cut into pieces)

- 1 lb of Brussels sprouts (trimmed and halved)

- 8 oz of small Yukon Gold potatoes, halved

- Cooking spray

Instructions

- Heat up oven to a temperature of 450°F.

- In a mixing bowl, whisk together 2 teaspoons vinegar, oil, mustard, thyme, salt, and pepper. Mix butternut squash, potatoes, parsnips and Brussels sprouts in a separate large bowl. Now add the mustard mixture to the squash mixture and toss together to coat.

- Line baking sheet with aluminum foil and coat with cooking spray. Then spread the vegetable mixture on it in a single layer. Bake in the preheated oven for about 35 minutes or until tender (Stir carefully using a spatula after 25 minutes). Remove pan from the oven after 35 minutes and drizzle the baked vegetable with the remaining 1 teaspoon vinegar; toss.

Spiced Apple Cranberry Sauce

Ingredients:

- 12 oz. of fresh cranberries (divided)

- ½ cup of packed light brown sugar

- ½ tsp of ground cinnamon

- ¼ tsp of ground cloves

- ¼ tsp of ground nutmeg

- 1 cup of chopped apple

- 4 tbsp of apple cider vinegar (divided)

- ½ tsp of kosher salt

- ½ tsp of black pepper

Instructions:

- Reserve ½ cup of cranberries. Prepare a saucepan, put the remaining cranberries in it together with the brown sugar and heat over medium-low. Add 2 ½ tbsp of cider vinegar, cloves, cinnamon and nutmeg to the cranberries and brown sugar in the saucepan.

Then cook for about 10 minutes while stirring frequently.

- Raise heat to medium-high. Stir in the chopped apple and the remaining vinegar. Cook for another 8 minutes. Stir in reserved cranberries, salt, and pepper

ACV Cucumber Salad

Ingredients:

- 1 tablespoon of cider vinegar

- 2 cups of sliced cucumbers

- 2 tbsp of chopped onions

- ½ cup of mayo

- Salt to taste

- Pepper to taste

Instructions

- Mix 2 cups of sliced cucumbers, 2 tablespoons chopped onions, ½ cup mayo, and 1 tbsp of apple cider vinegar in a mixing bowl. Then add salt and pepper to taste.

ACV Fire Cider

Ingredients:

- ½ cup of horseradish (peeled and diced)

- ½ cup of garlic (peeled and diced)

- ½ cup of onion (peeled and diced)

- ¼ cup of ginger (peeled and diced)

- ¼ cup of turmeric (peeled and diced)

- 1 habanero Chile (halved)

- 1 orange (quartered and thinly sliced crosswise)

- ½ lemon, quartered and thinly sliced crosswise

- ½ cup of chopped parsley

- 2 tbsp of chopped rosemary

- 2 tbsp of chopped thyme

- 1 tsp of black peppercorns

- 3 cups of raw unfiltered apple cider vinegar

- ¼ cup of raw honey

Instructions:

- Prepare a clean jar of about 1 quart; place all of the vegetables, fruits, herbs, and spices in the jar. Fill it with the cider vinegar, ensuring it covers all the contents in the jar. Also ensure that the jar is free of air bubbles, and then cap the jar. For jars with metal lid, place a piece of parchment or wax paper between the jar and the lid (this will help in preventing corrosion from the vinegar). After capping, shake well.

- Allow the jar to sit for about 3 to 6 weeks, shaking daily or every once in a while.

- Now strain the vinegar into a clean jar. Add as much honey as needed. Refrigerate until you are ready to use.

CHAPTER 3: APPLE CIDER VINEGAR DETOX AND SMOOTHIE

Lemon Water ACV Detox Drink

Ingredients:

- 1 cup of water

- 1 tablespoon of apple cider vinegar

- 1 tbsp of fresh lemon juice

- ½ tsp of ground cinnamon

- Pinch of cayenne pepper (optional)

- Honey (optional)

Instructions:

- Mix together all the ingredients in a glass. Add cayenne pepper and honey (if you desire) to make it sweeten the recipe.

Detox Cranberry Juice Drink

Ingredients:

- 1 tablespoon of apple cider vinegar

- ½ cup cranberry juice

- ¾ cup of water

- A splash of Lime Juice

Instructions:

- In a glass, combine all the ingredients.

- For more sweetness, add extra Lime Juice.

Apple Cider Vinegar Detox Smoothie

Ingredients:

- 1 tablespoon of apple cider vinegar

- ¼ cup of water

- 1 cup of apple (peeled and sliced)

- 2 tablespoons of avocado

- ¼ cup of ice

Instructions:

- Combine all the ingredients in a blender and puree

- Serve chilled.

ACV Green Tea Detox Drink

Ingredients:

- 1 cup of green tea

- 1 tablespoon apple cider vinegar

- Honey (to taste)

- Mint (to taste)

Instructions:

- Prepare the green tea. After that, add honey, mint and apple cider vinegar.

Cayenne and Sweet Lemon Detox Drink

Ingredients:

- 1 cup of water

- 1 tbsp of apple cider vinegar

- 1 tbsp of fresh lemon juice

- 1/8 tsp of cayenne pepper

- 1 tsp of honey

Instructions:

- Simply mix together all ingredients in a glass

- Serve and enjoy

Hot Apple Cider Vinegar Detox Drink

Ingredients:

- 2 cinnamon sticks

- 4 Cloves

- 1 ½ cups of water

- 2 tablespoon apple cider vinegar

- 2 tablespoon honey

- A lemon Slice (optional)

Instructions:

- Combine cinnamon, cloves, and water together in a pot and bring to a boil.

- Remove pot from the heat source and allow it to cool for about 30 minutes.

- Then add ACV, honey, and garnish with the lemon slice.

ACV Limeade Detox Drink

Ingredients:

- 1 cup of water

- 2 tablespoon of apple cider vinegar

- 6 tbsp of frozen limeade concentrate

- 1 lime wedge (optional)

- Mint leaves (optional)

Instructions:

- Combine all the ingredients together, serve in a glass and enjoy

Mixed Berries ACV Detox Smoothie

Ingredients:

- 1 cup of frozen mixed berries

- 1 banana

- 1 cup of almond milk

- 1/8 teaspoon vanilla extract

- 2 tablespoons of apple cider vinegar

- Pinch of salt

Instructions:

- Combine all the ingredients in a blender and blend. Add extra almond milk if it's too thick and needs to thin out a little.

Apple Pie Cinnamon Drink

Ingredients:

- 1 cup of water

- 2 tablespoons of cider vinegar

- 4 drops of liquid vanilla stevia

- 2 tablespoons of organic apple juice

- Dash of cinnamon

- 1-2 cubes of ice

Instructions:

- Combine all the ingredients in a cup and serve over ice

ACV Molasses Detox

Ingredients:

- 1 ½ cups water

- 2 tbsp of cider vinegar

- 2 tablespoons of blackstrap

Instructions:

- Simply mix all the ingredients together in a glass and enjoy.

CHAPTER 4: APPLE CIDER VINEGAR FOR HEALTH AND FIRST AID

Sunburn Relief

Ingredients:

- Water

- Apple cider vinegar

- Washcloth

Instructions:

- Take a shower using lukewarm to cool water to get any lotions or chemicals off your skin. Ensure not to use soap.

- Dry your body using a towel without irritating the sunburned skin. A padding motion is highly effective.

- Soak your washcloth/towel into the vinegar mixture (2 parts of cool water, 1 part of apple cider vinegar).

- Place the soaked towel onto your sunburned skin for 15minutes.

- Repeat regularly until the pain is reduced

Razor Bump Remedy

Ingredients:

- Apple cider vinegar

- Cotton ball

- Water

- Teabag

Instructions:

- Combine equal parts of apple cider vinegar and water together, and dab a cotton ball into the solution

- Apply the vinegar to the affected area and allow it to naturally dry

- Before the vinegar dries up, dip a black tea bag into a bowl of hot water for few minutes

- Remove the teabag from the hot water and refrigerate for about 10 minutes

- Massage the tea bag into the affected area for few minutes

- Repeat as many times as possible per day for quick relief

Bug Bite Treatment

Ingredients:

- 1 tsp of baking soda

- Water

- Apple cider vinegar

Instructions:

- Combine apple cider vinegar and water

- Dissolve a teaspoon of baking soda in water mixture and apply the paste on the affected area

- Leave it on for 10-20 minutes and then wash with lukewarm water.

Bruise Healer

Ingredients:

- Apple cider vinegar

- Water

- Washcloth

Instructions:

- Mix apple cider vinegar liquid with water in the ratio 2:1 (2 parts of the apple cider vinegar to 1 part of water)

- Soak a clean cloth in the solution and apply it on the affected area for 10-15 minutes

Stomach Upset Relief

Ingredients:

- 1 tbsp of apple cider vinegar

- 1 cup of warm water

- 1 tablespoon of honey

Instructions:

- Combine all ingredients and drink

Hiccups Relief

Ingredient:

- 1 cup of water

- 1 teaspoon of apple cider vinegar

Instructions:

- Add a teaspoonful of ACV to water and drink

Sore Throat Soother

Ingredients:

- ¼ cup of ACV

- ¼ cup of warm water

Instructions:

- Mix the ¼ cup of apple cider vinegar with the ¼ cup of warm water and gargle with it every hour

Bad Breath Remover

Ingredients:

- 2 tbsp of apple cider vinegar

- 1 cup of water

Instructions:

- Add two tablespoons of apple cider vinegar to 1 cup of water. Gargle for at least 30seconds before spitting it out

Stuffy Nose Treatment

Ingredients:

- 2 tsp of apple cider vinegar

- 1 cup of warm water

- 1 tbsp of honey (optional)

Instructions:

- Mix the apple cider vinegar with a cup of warm water and drink it at least three times per day

- Add a tablespoon of honey to the solution if desired.

Digestion Aid

Ingredients:

- 1 tsp of honey

- 1 tsp of apple cider vinegar

- 1 cup of warm water

Instructions:

- Mix the one teaspoon of honey and one teaspoon apple cider vinegar to a glass of warm water and drink it 30 minutes before mealtime.

Weight Reducer

Ingredients:

- 2 tbsp of apple cider vinegar

- A cup of water

Instructions

- Mix 2 tablespoons of ACV with water.

- Take at least 2-3 times per day or better still, drink it before every meal.

Energy Booster

Ingredients:

- Apple cider vinegar

- Water or a vegetable drink

Instructions

- Add 1 or 2 tablespoons of ACV to a glass chilled vegetable drink or to a glass of water. Drink to boost energy

Appetite and Cholesterol Reduction

Ingredients:

- 30 ml of apple cider vinegar

- Water (about 500 ml)

Instructions:

- Dilute 30 ml of apple cider vinegar in about 500mL of water and drink it every day for 12 weeks

Nighttime Leg Cramps

Ingredients:

- 2 tbsp of apple cider vinegar

- 1 tsp of honey

- Water

Instructions:

- Mix the apple cider vinegar with one teaspoon of honey in a glass of warm water

- Drink to relieve the nighttime leg cramps.

Teeth whitener

Ingredients:

- 1 cup of water

- 2 tbsp apple cider vinegar

Instructions:

- Gargle with the mix in the morning

- Brush as usual after gargle

All-Natural Cleansing Products

Ingredients:

- ¼ cup of apple cider vinegar

- Water

Instructions:

- Add ¼ cup of ACV to a 12 or 16 ounce-spray bottle filled with water

- The vinegar scent dissipates after a few minutes of use, leaving a naturally clean home.

All-Natural Fruit and Vegetables Wash

Ingredients:

- 1 ½ cups of water,

- ¾ cup of ACV

- 1 tablespoon baking soda

- 10 drops of lemon essential oil

Instructions:

- Get a 16 ounce glass spray bottle; add all the ingredients together in the bottle. Cover/cap the bottle and mix together by shaking gently

- Cap bottle and shake gently to mix well.

- Ready to be used for washing vegetables and fruit.

Dandruff Remover

Ingredients:

- ¼ cup of apple cider vinegar

- ¼ cup of water

Instructions:

- Mix the ingredients together in a spray bottle

- Spritz the mix on your scalp and wrap your head in a towel. Leave for about 30 – 60 minutes

- Wash your hair as usual

Cancer Prevention

Ingredients:

- Apple cider vinegar

Instructions:

- Incorporate the ACV into your diet by using it for cooking or dilute apple cider vinegar into water and drink as a beverage (1-2 tablespoons mixed in a large glass of water)

CHAPTER 5: APPLE CIDER VINEGAR FOR BEAUTY

Detox Ginger bath

Ingredients:

- 1 cup of apple cider vinegar

- 1/3 cup of baking soda (optional)

- 1/3 cup of Epsom salt

- 1/3 cup of sea salt

- 3 tbsp of ground ginger

- Water

Instructions:

- Mix all the ingredients together except for the ACV, add the baking soda if desired.

- Pour the mixture in a warm bath and add 1 cup of ACV as the bath fills

- Soak for up to 30 minutes and ensure you drink lots of water while soaking. Get out of the bathroom if you start to feel uncomfortable.

- Dry your body immediately after leaving the bathroom.

Ensure to drink water before, during, and after bathing to replenish fluid intake.

Acne remedy

Ingredients:

- Apple cider vinegar

- Cotton ball

- Water (warm)

Instructions:

- In a mixing bowl, combine raw and unfiltered ACV with filtered water.

- Dab a cotton ball in the solution and apply it on the area of the skin that is affected.

- Leave it for about 10 - 12 minutes and then rinse it off using warm water.

Apple Cider Vinegar Facial Toner

Ingredients:

- Apple Cider Vinegar (raw)

- Filtered water

- Lavender essential oil (if desired)

Instructions:

- Combine 1 part of apple cider vinegar with 4 parts of filtered water (for sensitive skin)

- Combine 1 part of apple cider vinegar with 2 parts of filtered water (for dry or normal skin)

- Combine 1 part of apple cider vinegar with 1 part of water (for oily skin)

- If adding lavender essential oil, use about 2 – 3 drops for every 8 ounces of toner

- Leave it for a few minutes before rinsing it off with cold water.

Skin Soother

Instructions:

- Pour some ACV in a bathtub of warm water.

- Soak in the tub for 15-20 minutes.

- Allow the protective acid to soak into your skin and ensure to follow this routine to maintain the pH levels of your skin.

Spots and Wrinkles Remover

Ingredients:

- Water

- ACV

Instructions:

- Mix 2 parts water with 1-part ACV. Dab a little of the mix on a cotton ball and use it on the age spot and wrinkles.

- Leave it for about 15 minutes and then rinse it off with cold water.

Foot deodorizer

Ingredients:

- 1 cup of ACV

- 4 cups of water

Instructions:

- Get a sizable bowl and mix 1 cup of apple cider vinegar with 4 cups water in it

- Soak feet for 15 minutes in the bowl

- Then rinse and dry.

Deep Pore Detoxifying Treatment Mask

Ingredients:

- Apple cider vinegar

- Honey

- Green clay

Instructions:

- Mix equal parts of apple cider vinegar and green clay or fuller's earth

- Add 1 tsp of honey to it. Apply this on the skin and leave for about 10 – 15 minutes.

(Make use of less Apple Cider Vinegar if your skin is sensitive)

ACV Eczema Remedy

Ingredients:

- 1 tbsp of apple cider vinegar

- 1 pint of water

Instructions:

- Spray the affected area with the ingredient mixture or use as a bath rinse

ACV Dandruff Remedy

Ingredients:

- 1 pint of water

- 1 tbsp of apple cider vinegar

Instructions:

- Combine the ingredients and create a bath rinse with the combination

Quick ACV Facemask

Ingredients:

- 1 tablespoon of Apple Cider Vinegar
- 2 tablespoons of honey

Instructions:

- Mix 2 tbsp of honey with 1 tbsp of apple cider vinegar. Clean your face, apply the mixture on your face and leave for about 20 minutes.
- Then rinse with lukewarm water followed by a fresh rinse.

Foot Soak for Rough Skin

Ingredients:

- Apple Cider Vinegar
- Water

Instructions:

- Soak your feet in equal parts of warm water and apple cider vinegar mixed together, to soften up dry and tough skin.

- Soak it for about 30 minutes to one hour to get rid of stubborn calluses, and then shed off with a buffer.

ACV Face Pack

Ingredients:

- 1 tsp Arrowroot

- 1 tsp Dabur Gulabari Rose Water

- ¼ tsp Apple cider vinegar

- ¼ tsp Nutritional yeast

- 1 tsp ginger

Instructions:

- Combine 1 tsp of arrowroot, 1 tsp of rosewater, ¼ tsp of apple cider vinegar, ¼ tsp of nutritional yeast and 1 tsp of ginger in a bowl

- Apply it to your face.

- Rinse with warm water and pat dry

ACV Hair Care

Ingredients:

- 1/3 cup of Apple Cider Vinegar

- Shampoo

Instructions:

- Shampoo your hair and soak with 1/3 cup of ACV

- Rinse afterward

Skin Exfoliation

Ingredients:

- Apple Cider Vinegar

- Warm water

Instructions:

- Pour some apple cider vinegar in a bathtub of warm water and stay in the tub for 15-20 minutes.

- Allow the protective acid to soak into your skin.

ACV for Psoriasis

Ingredients:

- Apple Cider Vinegar

- Water

Instructions:

- Add 1 part of apple cider vinegar to 3 parts of lukewarm water.

- Use on the affected area using a washcloth for about 1 hour30 minutes

Dark Armpits Lightening

Ingredients:

- Apple Cider Vinegar

- Water

- Cotton pads

Instructions:

- Mix equal parts of water and ACV together in a mixing bowl.

- Soak about 2 cotton pads and use on each underarm like a sheet mask.

- Leave for about 15-20 minutes before rinsing with water.

Armpit Detox

Ingredients:

- 1 tbsp of Bentonite clay

- ½ tbsp of Apple Cider Vinegar

Instructions:

- Mix all the ingredients together until the mixture becomes a paste.

- Apply the mix on clean armpits and leave for about 15-20 minutes or until dry.

- Then wash off and pat dry.

Cellulite Remover

Ingredients:

- Apple Cider Vinegar

- Water

- Honey

Instructions:

- Mix 1 part of the Apple Cider Vinegar to 2 parts of water

- Add a drop of honey and scrub it on the part of the body that is affected.

CHAPTER 6: APPLE CIDER VINEGAR FOR HOME AND CLEANING

Jar Sanitizer

Ingredients:

- Apple cider vinegar

- Soapy Water

Instructions:

- Add 1 part of apple cider vinegar to 1 part of warm soapy water. Scrub well with the solution to disinfect your jars.

Kettle Cleaner

Ingredients:

- 3 cups of Apple cider vinegar

- Water

Instructions:

- Boil the ingredients in the tea kettle for about 5 minutes and allow to sit overnight before rinsing with water

ACV Pots/ Pans Cleaner

Ingredients:

- Salt

- Cornstarch or Flour

- Apple cider vinegar

Instructions:

- Dilute equal parts of salt and cornstarch with sufficient vinegar to make a paste.

- Use it to scrub off sticky foods from the pots.

Coffeemaker Cleaner

Ingredients:

- Apple cider vinegar

- Water

Instructions:

- Add two parts of the Apple cider vinegar to 1 part of water

- Pour into the coffeemaker and then run a normal brew cycle

Apple Cider Vinegar Silver, Copper & Bronze Polish

Ingredients:

- ¼ cup of apple cider

- ¼ cup of table salt

- ¼ cup of citrus oil

Instructions:

- Whisk all the ingredients together.

- Then rub on silver, bronze, or copper and buff gently until tarnish is removed.

Sticker Removal

Ingredients:

- Apple Cider Vinegar

Instructions:

- Soak the stickers in apple cider vinegar for about 20 minutes

- Remove and scrape off with a butter knife

ACV Fridge Cleaner

Ingredients:

- 1 cup of Apple cider vinegar

- 1 cup of Water

- 10 drops of essential oils

Instructions:

- Mix all ingredients together.

- Transfer into a spray bottle

- To use, spray on refrigerator surfaces and wipe down.

Apple Cider Vinegar Flycatcher

Ingredients:

- ½ cup apple cider vinegar

- 3-4 drops dish soap

- 5 drops grapefruit essential oil

Instructions:

- Gently mix all the ingredients together

- Place next to the fruit bowl and leave it for 24 hours to catch fruit flies.

Stain Removal from Dishes

Ingredients:

- Apple cider vinegar

- Salt

Instructions:

- Scrub the dishes with 1 part of apple cider vinegar and 1 part of the salt

To Clean Carpet/Rugs

Ingredients:

- Apple cider vinegar

- Water

Instructions:

- Spray carpet or rug with a solution mix of apple vinegar and water.

- Leave the rug for about 60 minutes before vacuuming

Yellow Clothing Stains

Ingredients:

- Warm Water

- Apple cider vinegar

Instructions:

- Soak the clothing in a solution of vinegar and warm water (12 parts of warm water to 1 part of vinegar) overnight before washing

Wrinkle removal from Clothes

Ingredients:

- Apple cider vinegar

- Water

Instructions:

- Add 3 parts of water to 1 part of vinegar and transfer into a spray bottle

- Spray the mix on the wrinkles and allow the clothes to hang dry

Candle wax removal

Ingredients:

- Apple cider vinegar

- Water

- Hairdryer

Instructions:

- Heat the pile wax with a hairdryer and soak up as much of it as you can with a rag.

- Use a 1:1 ratio mixture of vinegar and water (1 part of water to 1 part of vinegar) to remove the rest.

Ink stains removal

Ingredients:

- Apple cider vinegar

Instruction:

- Apply full-strength vinegar to a clean cloth

- Wipe the stain with the cloth until stain is removed

Unclog Drains

Ingredients:

- ½ cup of baking soda

- 1 cup of vinegar

Instructions:

- Combine the ingredients and pour into your drain

Washing machine Cleaner

Ingredients:

- 2 cups of ACV

Instruction:

- Pour the 2 cups of vinegar into the washing machine and run a full cycle without any clothes in it

Apple Cider Vinegar Drain Freshener

Ingredients:

- ¼ cup baking soda

- ½ cup of apple cider vinegar

- 1 cup of hot water

- 5-6 drops of lemon essential oil

Instructions:

- Pour the baking soda down any clogged drain.

- Now combine lemon oil and cider vinegar together.

- Gently pour down the drain and allow it to sit and foam for about 20-30 minutes before rinsing with 1-2 cups of hot water.

Remove Mildew from Bathtubs

Ingredients:

- Apple cider vinegar

- Water

- Lemon essential oil (optional)

Instructions:

- Use a mixture of 1 part of water and 1 part of vinegar for lighter stains and give full strength attention for heavy mildew. Add essential oil for a fresh scent, if desired.

All-Purpose Vinegar Cleaning Scrub

Ingredients

- 1/2 cup baking soda

- 1/4 cup vinegar

- 5-10 drops citrus or lavender essential oils

Instructions:

- Stir all the ingredients together.

- Apply using a scrub brush and wash clean using warm water.

Apple Cider Vinegar Wood Polish

Ingredients:

- ½ cup of cider vinegar

- ½ cup of olive oil

- 20-30 drops of lemon or orange essential oil

Instructions:

- Combine all ingredients and transfer into a spray bottle.

To use, spray on wood and wipe clean.

CHAPTER 7: APPLE CIDER VINEGAR

FOR PETS

ACV Flea and Tick Remedy

Ingredients:

- 8 ounces of ACV

- 4 ounces of warm water

- ½ teaspoon of salt

- ½ tsp of baking soda

Instructions:

- Put the dry ingredients into a spray bottle and then slowly add the liquids. It is best to do this over a sink. Store it in a cool, dark place.

- This spray may necessarily not kill fleas and ticks, but it will keep them away from your dog as long as you treat your dog(s) regularly.

ACV for Itchy Skin

Ingredients:

- 1 tbsp of apple cider vinegar

- 1 pint of water

Instructions:

- Combine the ingredients and rinse your dog with the mix after bathing the dog

ACV Ear Infection Remedy

Ingredients:

- Apple cider vinegar

- Water

- Cotton ball

Instructions:

- Combine together, equal parts of water and vinegar.

- Apply 5 ml of the solution to the dog's ear and wipe the inside using a cotton ball

ACV Hot Spots Remedy

Ingredients:

- Apple cider vinegar

- Water

- Cotton ball

Instructions:

- Mix equal parts of water and apple cider vinegar in a bowl

- Soak a cotton ball in the mix and dab it on the hot spot

ACV Pet Odor Removal

Ingredients:

- 1 tablespoon of apple cider vinegar

- 1 pint of water

Instruction:

- Combine the ingredients and pour over your pet after bathing

Irritated Paws Reliever

Ingredients:

- Apple cider vinegar

- Water

Instructions:

- Soothe the irritation by soaking your pup's paws in 2:1 water to vinegar mixture for about 5 minutes.

Pet Immunity Boost

Ingredients:

- Apple cider vinegar

Instructions:

- Add the apple cider vinegar to your pet's food or water for the improved immune system. Use one teaspoon ACV for small dogs, two teaspoons ACV for medium-sized dogs and one tablespoon ACV for large dogs

ACV Fungal infections Remedy

Ingredients:

- Apple cider vinegar

- Water

Instruction:

- Apply an equal part mixture of ACV and water (50:50) to the affected area.

CHAPTER; 8 APPLE CIDER VINEGAR FOR WEIGHT LOSS

Apple Cider Vinegar with Honey

Ingredients:

- 1 tsp of ACV
- 2 tsp of honey
- 1 cup of warm water

Instructions:

- Mix the apple cider vinegar and honey together in a glass of warm water.
- Stir and drink.

Apple Cider Vinegar and Cinnamon

Ingredients:

- 1 tsp of apple cider vinegar

- ½ tsp of Ceylon cinnamon powder

- 1 cup of water

Instructions:

- Add the cinnamon powder and the water to a pot and boil it.

- After boiling, allow it to cool then add ACV to the solution in the pot.

- Stir together well and drink.

Apple Cider Vinegar and Fenugreek Seeds

Ingredients:

- 1 tsp of ACV

- 2 tsp of fenugreek seeds

- 1 cup of water

Instructions:

- Preferably soak the fenugreek seeds overnight in a cup filled with water.

- Add ACV (about 1 teaspoon) to the fenugreek water the next morning.

- Stir together and drink.

Apple Cider Vinegar and Green Tea

Ingredients:

- 1 tsp of ACV

- 1 tsp of green tea leaves

- 1 tsp of honey

- 1 cup of water

Instructions:

- Prepare a pot and heat the cup of water in it until the water just starts to boil.

- Remove the pot from the heat source and stir in the green tea leaves. Close the lid and allow it to steep for about 3 minutes.

- After, strain the tea into a cup and add the ACV and honey

- Then mix well and drink.

Apple Cider Vinegar Salad Dressing

Ingredients:

- 2 tsp of ACV

- 4 tsp of extra virgin olive oil

- 1 tsp of Dijon mustard

- ½ tsp of lemon zest

- ¼ tsp of freshly ground black pepper

- 1 tbsp of chopped fresh herbs

- Salt to taste

Instructions:

- Toss all the ingredients into a glass jar and shake the jar well.

- Drizzle the mixture all over a healthy and crunchy salad.

Apple Cider Vinegar Healthy Smoothie

Ingredients:

- 1 tsp of ACV

- ½ cup of pomegranate

- 1 tsp of chopped apricot

- A bunch of baby spinach

Instructions:

- Combine all the ingredients together in a blender and blend.

- Pour the blended mix into a glass and drink.

Apple Cider Vinegar Drink

Ingredients:

- Ice

- 1 cup of filtered water

- 2 tsp of raw apple cider vinegar (with mother)

- 2 tsp of lemon juice fresh

- Liquid stevia to taste

- fresh berries and mint leaves (if desired)

Instructions:

- Add the ice, filtered water, apple cider vinegar, and lemon juice to a glass. Add the liquid stevia to sweeten the mix to the desired taste.

- Stir and drink.

- If desired, add fresh ginger, honey or maple syrup, fresh fruit or the juice of thawed berries, or a splash of natural 100% fruit juice for extra flavor.

ACV Lemon Water Drink

Ingredients:

- 1 cup of water

- 1 tablespoon apple cider vinegar

- 1 tablespoon fresh lemon juice

- ½ teaspoon ground cinnamon

- 1 pinch cayenne pepper (optional)

- Honey (optional)

Instruction:

- Combine all the ingredients in a glass. Add extra honey if desired to make it sweeter.

- Enjoy!

ACV Cranberry Juice Drink

Ingredients:

- 1 tablespoon of apple cider vinegar

- 1/2 cup of cranberry juice

- 1 tablespoon of honey

- Splash of lime juice

- 3/4 cup of water

Instructions:

- Mix all the ingredients together in a glass. (For more sweetness, add extra lime juice).

CONCLUSION

Apple cider vinegar, like all other kinds of vinegar, is quite acidic. This means that attention should be given to the rate and volume of consumption of ACV. While there are several health benefits derived from taking the apple cider vinegar, consuming too much of it (especially undiluted) can cause unwanted adverse effects. It is important then to ensure that the vinegar is diluted, especially when applying it on the affected skin. A safe way of drinking vinegar is drinking it with the help of a straw, as this will help prevent unnecessary and prolonged acidic contact with the teeth. In conclusion, ACV is a good natural remedy for numerous ailments. However, basic factors such as the user's age and health condition should be considered when using apple cider vinegar.